SOMATIC EXERCISE
FOR BEGINNERS

A Gentle Path to Pain Relief and Wellness

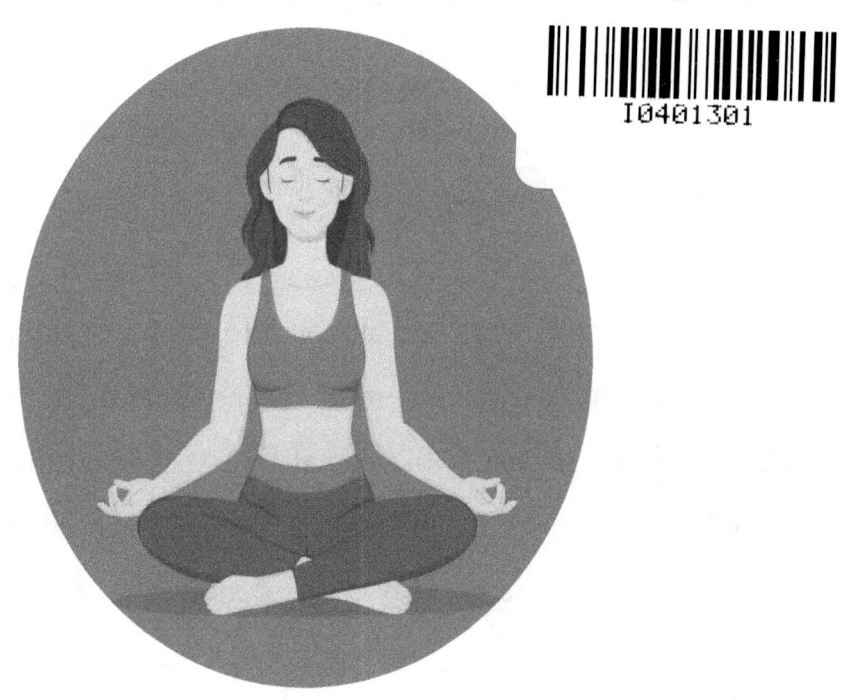

Gary B. Flanagan

Copyright © 2024 by Gary B. Flanagan

All rights reserved. No part of this publication may be reproduced, stored in a retrieval system, or transmitted in any form or by any means, electronic, mechanical, photocopying, recording, or otherwise, without the prior written permission of the copyright owner, except for brief quotations in critical reviews and certain other noncommercial uses permitted by copyright law.

Declaimer

This book is a work of nonfiction. Names, characters, places, and incidents are either the product of the author's imagination are used fictitiously. Any resemblance to actual persons, living or dead, business establishments, events, or locales is entirely coincidental

ABOUT THE AUTHOR

I am a seasoned life and fitness mentor with a wealth of experience in both fitness and psychology. Having personally triumphed over challenges with low self-esteem through self-development and exercise, my journey inspired me to dedicate my career to helping others. With a deep understanding of attitudes toward failure and resilience, I combine fitness and psychological principles to offer a unique and effective approach to personal growth. My compassionate and relatable guidance has empowered countless individuals to transform their mindsets, unlock their full potential, and embrace a life of confidence and success. My unwavering commitment to my client's well-being makes me a trusted partner on their journey to self-improvement.

TABLE OF CONTENTS

ABOUT THE AUTHOR 3

TABLE OF CONTENTS 4

OVERVIEW OF THE BOOK 7

INTRODUCTIONS 9

CHAPTER 1 11

   Starting Your Somatic Journey 11

   What are Somatic Exercises? 13

   Benefits for Body and Mind 14

   Understanding the Foundations 16

CHAPTER 2 18

   The History and Evolution of Somatic Practices 18

   Origins of Somatic Exercises 21

   Key Figures and Pioneers 22

   Milestones in the Development of Somatic Practices ... 24

CHAPTER 3 27

   The Science Behind Somatic Exercises 27

Understanding the Mind-Body Connection 28

Research and Evidence 30

The Neuroscience of Movement and Awareness 31

Practical Application 33

CHAPTER 4 35

Basic Somatic Exercises 36

Preparing for Practice 39

Essential Warm-Up Exercises 41

Beginner-Friendly Somatic Movements 42

CHAPTER 5 45

Targeting Common Problem Areas. 45

Relieving back pain 45

Improving posture 48

Enhancing flexibility 53

Reducing tension in the neck and shoulders 55

Somatic strategies for stress reduction 58

Applying awareness to household chores 60

Somatic principles for walking and running............61

Mindful sitting and standing...............................63

CHAPTER 6...66

Overcoming Common Challenges.......................66

Addressing Common Beginner Mistakes 68

Tips for Consistency and Motivation 70

Modifications for Different Fitness Levels 72

CHAPTER 7...75

Integrating Somatic Awareness into Daily Life 75

Tracking Progress and Setting Goals..............77

Setting SMART Goals for Your Somatic Practice........80

Tracking Your Progress and Celebrating Milestones....82

Expanding Your Knowledge 83

Conclusion...85

OVERVIEW OF THE BOOK

Welcome to Somatic Exercises for Beginners, your guide to a transforming journey through body awareness and mindful movement. This book is intended to introduce you to the realm of somatics, a novel method of training that goes beyond physical conditioning. Here, you'll find a practice that focuses on reconnecting with your body, developing self-care skills, and discovering gentle movement solutions to everyday problems.

What sets Somatic Exercises apart? Unlike standard fitness routines, somatics focuses on the mind-body connection. We'll look at easy strategies to improve your body awareness, allowing you to move more intentionally and easily. Whether you're a complete novice or want to improve your understanding of movement, this book offers a safe and supportive environment to discover the benefits of somatics.

What you will discover inside:

- **The Fundamentals of Somatics:** We'll go over the fundamentals of somatics, discussing how it may improve your health and solve common issues such as stress, back discomfort, and bad posture.
- **Connecting with Your Body**: Discover easy strategies for mindfulness and body awareness to provide the groundwork for your somatic practice.

- **Gentle Movement for Everyday Life**: Learn about a range of somatic exercises that target specific difficulties, such as relaxation, posture improvement, and pain reduction.
- **Exploring various somatic practices**: Get an overview of popular somatic methods such as the Feldenkrais Method and the Alexander Technique.
- **Personalizing Your Journey**: Learn how to tailor exercises to your specific requirements and establish a long-term somatic practice that fits easily into your everyday routine.
- **Setting objectives and Tracking Progress**: We'll provide you with resources to help you create objectives, measure your progress, and celebrate your accomplishments along the road.

Somatic Exercises for Beginners invites you to rediscover the joy of movement and develop a deeper connection with your body. By implementing these gentle activities into your daily routine, you'll find yourself moving more freely, lowering tension, and cultivating a sense of general well-being. Let us begin!

INTRODUCTIONS

Have you ever experienced a sense of unfamiliarity with your own body? Have you ever felt like your body is unfamiliar to you? Perhaps you wake up with a crick in your neck after a long day slumped over a computer, or your lower back hurts after chasing your kids around the park. You are not alone. In today's fast-paced society, getting disconnected from our bodies is easy, resulting in tension, discomfort, and a general sense of unease.

What if there was a way to reconnect with your body, not just through exercise, but through conscious movement? This is where Somatic Exercises come in. Forget the push-ups and crunches (unless you enjoy them!). Somatics is a peaceful and uplifting practice that helps you rediscover the joy of movement while also providing relief from common aches and pains. Consider feeling secure and comfortable in your own skin. Imagine being able to bend down to pick something up without wincing, or walking for kilometers without feeling as if your legs are ready to fail. Somatics can help you do this.

Here is a little glimpse of what you may expect:

- **Tame the Tension:** Do your neck and shoulders feel like battlegrounds after a long day? Somatics provides specific activities to relieve tension and discomfort.
- **Back to bliss**: Say goodbye to your annoying backache! Somatics can help you discover the source of your discomfort and guide you

through gentle movements that promote healing and avoid future issues.

- **Posture Power:** Forget slouching! Somatics teaches you how to maintain a strong and aligned posture, which boosts your confidence and lowers the strain on your body.
- **Flexibility for Freedom:** Do you want to touch your toes without feeling like you're going to snap in half? Somatics takes you on a journey of enhanced flexibility, allowing you to move more freely and experience a broader range of motion.
- **Stress Less, Move More:** Feeling overwhelmed? Somatics provides effective stress and anxiety reduction techniques based on mindful movement and body awareness.
- **Mindful Movement in Everyday Life:** Somatics involves more than just mat exercises. Learn how to incorporate mindful movement concepts into everyday tasks such as sitting, standing, walking, jogging, and even domestic chores!

Somatics is more than just exercise; it's a conversation with your own body. Imagine yourself moving with purpose, grounded, and present in the moment. This book will help you start that conversation and rediscover your incredible potential.

Are you ready to go on this adventure of mindful movement and self-discovery? Let us begin!

CHAPTER 1

Starting Your Somatic Journey

Welcome to the somatic adventure! This is your chance to truly connect with your body and mind in a manner that typical workouts may not allow. Think of somatic exercises as a means to communicate with your inner self, concentrating on how you feel from the inside out. This method makes your body feel better and promotes mental clarity and emotional peace.

Understanding Somatic Exercises.

Imagine mild motions that help you become more aware of your body and its sensations. These exercises retrain your nervous system, allowing you to relax, improve your posture, and boost your mobility. Moving thoughtfully makes it simpler to move without strain, reducing the chance of injury and improving general physical function.

Benefits for Beginners

You'll notice some significant advantages right away. Somatic activities can help relieve chronic pain, lower tension, and enhance coordination and balance. Paying attention to how your body feels throughout each exercise will help you acquire a better understanding of your movement patterns, leading to long-term positive improvements.

Getting Started

To begin your somatic practice, select a peaceful, comfortable location where you will not be interrupted. Wear loose, comfortable clothing that allows you to move freely. Begin with easy exercises to ease you into somatic movement. These might include gentle stretches, slow, deliberate motions, and concentrated breathing exercises.

Setting Expectations

Keep in mind that progress here is determined by your ability to focus and be alert rather than your pace. Take your time with each exercise, focusing on how your body feels. Patience is essential—do not rush. Enjoy the procedure and pay attention to your body's feedback.

Setting a Routine

Consistency is your best friend. Try to practice every day, even if it's only for a few minutes. Over time, you should notice changes in your posture, flexibility, and overall well-being.

Starting your somatic journey entails more than just performing physical activities. It's about developing a greater appreciation for and knowledge of your own body. This thoughtful exercise benefits both your physical and mental health, enabling you to live a balanced and peaceful existence. Enjoy your adventure!

What are Somatic Exercises?

Imagine a world where exercise is more than just pushing yourself but also about reconnecting with your body. That is the miracle of somatic exercises! Unlike standard routines, Somatics emphasizes the mind-body connection. It's about becoming more aware of your body's feelings, which will help you to move more purposefully and quickly. Somatic Exercises are gentle interactions with your body. Simple motions and stretches will teach you how to release tension in troubled areas such as your neck and shoulders and identify the source of your bothersome back discomfort.

However, Somatics extends beyond treating particular ailments. It's about developing a strong, aligned posture that improves confidence while reducing pressure on your body. Imagine touching your toes without feeling like you're about to snap in half! Somatic exercises lead to enhanced flexibility, allowing you to move more easily and freely. Somatics' beauty stems from its adaptability. You may apply mindful movement ideas to your daily life. Learn to sit and stand mindfully, turning basic tasks like folding laundry into chances for gentle movement. Somatics is more than simply bodily well-being. It enables you to handle stress and anxiety. By being more aware of your body's feelings, you may learn to relax and quiet your nervous system, resulting in a better overall sense of well-being.

Benefits for Body and Mind

Consider a world where exercise not only enhances your body but also relaxes your mind. That is the wonder of Somatic Exercises! Unlike typical workouts that are only focused on developing muscle or burning calories, Somatics takes a comprehensive approach that benefits both your physical and emotional health.

Physical Advantages

- Reduced Tension and Pain: Does your neck resemble a battlefield after a long day? Somatic exercises target specific parts of the body, such as the neck and shoulders, reducing tension and encouraging relaxation. Back discomfort can be eliminated as well. Somatic movements aid in identifying the underlying problem, such as bad posture or weak core muscles, and addressing it with gentle stretches and exercises, resulting in healing and preventing future disorders.
- Improved posture: Say goodbye to slouching! Somatic exercises show you how to develop a strong and aligned posture. This not only enhances your confidence but also decreases tension in your body, which improves your general health.
- Improved Flexibility: Have you ever wished you could get back to touching your toes? Somatic motions will take you on a trip toward greater flexibility. You may achieve a wider range of motion by gently stretching and moving your body with

awareness, allowing you to move more freely and enjoy everyday activities more.

Benefits for the Mind

Somatics is more than simply physical movement; it's also an effective stress and anxiety management technique. You'll learn to relax and soothe your nervous system with mindful movement and body awareness practices. This results in a stronger sense of well-being, helping you to confront daily problems with a clearer head.

- Body Awareness: Somatic exercises help you become more conscious of your body's sensations. This increased awareness helps you to connect with your body on a deeper level, cultivating self-compassion and gratitude for your physical vessel.
- Improved Focus and Presence: Somatics' attentive feature helps you become more present in the moment. By concentrating on your body's motions and feelings, you may calm your mind and increase your general focus and attention, both during and after your practice.

Somatic Exercises have a knock-on effect, relieving bodily aches and pains while also boosting mental serenity and well-being. This all-encompassing approach to movement helps you feel more comfortable and secure in your own skin, both physically and psychologically.

Understanding the Foundations

Understanding the fundamentals of somatic exercises is vital for novices to completely appreciate the advantages and principles of this practice. At its foundation, somatic exercise stresses the mind-body connection, concentrating on interior experiences rather than exterior performance. This technique helps build a profound awareness of how your body moves and feels.

Mind-Body Connection: The cornerstone of somatic exercises resides in the mind-body connection. By paying great attention to your body's feelings, you learn to recognize and release tension, enhance movement efficiency, and promote overall physical well-being. This attentive method helps retrain the nervous system, creating new, healthier movement habits.

Historical Context: Somatic techniques have evolved over decades, influenced by pioneers like Thomas Hanna, who created the word "somatics." Understanding the historical background helps you grasp the evolution and refining of these strategies. Knowing the roots and major personalities helps increase your appreciation and devotion to the practice.

Scientific Basis: Research shows that somatic workouts improve physical and mental well-being. According to studies, these exercises can help with chronic pain, flexibility, and stress management.

Understanding the scientific basis can help you feel more secure about adopting somatic workouts into your practice.

Understanding these fundamental concepts, you'll be better prepared to begin your somatic journey, making your practice more efficient and fulfilling.

> "It's not just exercise, it's self-discovery. Somatic Exercise for Beginners empowers you to move with intention, breathe with freedom, and rediscover the joy of being in your body."

CHAPTER 2

The History and Evolution of Somatic Practices

Somatic practices, which focus on integrating the mind and body to improve movement and awareness, have a long and varied history. These techniques have emerged as a result of contributions from various major personalities and movements, each of which has added depth and insight to the area.

Early Foundations: Somatic practices have their roots in ancient societies where movement and body awareness were central to everyday living and spiritual rituals. Yoga and Tai Chi, for example, are ancient disciplines that involve mindfulness and body awareness, which are essential components of somatic activities. The formalization of somatic practices began in the late nineteenth and early twentieth century, with the introduction of methodologies like the Alexander Technique and the Feldenkrais Method.

The Alexander Technique, developed by F.M. Alexander, focuses on improving posture and movement efficiency in order to relieve tension and improve general well-being. Alexander, an Australian actor, developed the approach after resolving his own voice and breathing issues through better body alignment and movement patterns. The strategy helps people to become more conscious of their behaviors and make deliberate adjustments to improve their physical function.

The Feldenkrais approach: Named after its originator, Moshe Feldenkrais, this approach focuses on learning via movement. Feldenkrais, a physicist and judo specialist, created his technique following a knee injury. He utilized his expertise of anatomy, physics, and martial arts to develop a system for improving people's mobility and self-awareness. The Feldenkrais Method employs gentle, exploratory movements to assist people in discovering more efficient and pain-free ways of moving.

Mid-twentieth century: Several additional notable somatic techniques emerged during this time period.

Ida Rolf developed Rolfing Structural Integration, which focuses on balancing the body in the gravitational field through deep tissue manipulation and movement teaching. Rolf thought that by adjusting the body's alignment, one could relieve chronic pain and enhance general function. Rudolf Laban developed Laban Movement Analysis, which gives a framework for monitoring, describing, and analyzing human movement. It is commonly utilized in dance, physical therapy, and other disciplines to improve movement efficiency and expressiveness.

Late twentieth century: Thomas Hanna invented the word "somatics" in the 1970s. Hanna, a philosopher and movement instructor, introduced the phrase to describe techniques that emphasize the body as perceived from within. His research stressed the nervous system's involvement in determining movement patterns and pioneered the notion of "somatic education," which seeks to retrain the nervous system to enhance mobility and minimize discomfort.

Contemporary Developments: Somatic practices have evolved over the last few decades, embracing new research and approaches from neurology, psychology, and biomechanics. Modern somatic techniques frequently stress a comprehensive approach that includes physical, emotional, and cognitive elements of well-being.

Mindfulness-Based Somatic Practices: These practices, including Body-Mind Centering and Somatic Experiencing, use mindfulness and body awareness to support healing and personal growth. They highlight the significance of listening to the body's messages and employing movement to relieve stress and trauma.

Scientific Validation: Many somatic techniques have been scientifically validated by recent studies. According to research, somatic exercises can improve physical function, alleviate chronic pain, and improve mental wellness. This scientific basis has contributed to the acceptability and popularity of somatic techniques in mainstream health and wellness circles. Why Is Somatic History Important?

Understanding Somatics' history allows us to comprehend the practice's richness and complexity. It demonstrates how many concepts and methodologies have come together to become the Somatics we know today. By appreciating its origins, we may feel linked to a long line of practitioners who have investigated the potential of mindful movement for self-discovery and well-being.

As you engage on your Somatic journey, keep in mind that you are not simply exercising; you are also tapping into a rich tradition of conscious movement techniques that have benefited people for decades. Enjoy your exploration!

Origins of Somatic Exercises

Somatic exercises have their roots in ancient techniques that stressed mental and physical harmony. Early inspirations include disciplines such as yoga and Tai Chi, which have been practiced for thousands of years and combine mindfulness and physical movement to improve overall wellness.

The formalization of somatic practices began in the late nineteenth and early twentieth century, with the creation of particular strategies for increasing body awareness and movement efficiency. F.M. Alexander, an Australian actor, developed the Alexander Technique after resolving his own voice and breathing issues with better body alignment and movement. His technique aims to reduce stress and improve general physical function by raising awareness of habitual movement patterns.

Around the same period, Moshe Feldenkrais, a physicist and judo specialist, created the Feldenkrais Method. Following a knee injury, Feldenkrais used his understanding of anatomy, physics, and martial arts to develop a method that employs gentle, exploratory motions to retrain the nervous system, resulting in more efficient and less painful movement.

These pioneering efforts paved the way for current somatic exercises, stressing the significance of interior sensations and the mind-body link. Understanding these roots allows novices to comprehend the scope and historical context of their somatic practice.

Key Figures and Pioneers

Several major personalities and pioneers have made substantial contributions to the development of somatic exercises, including core methodologies and ideologies. Understanding their contributions adds vital context to the approaches we use today.

F.M. Alexander (1869-1955): Frederick Matthias Alexander, an Australian actor, created the Alexander Technique in the early twentieth century. After having recurrent voice problems, Alexander learned that improper posture and movement patterns were to blame. His approach focuses on increasing body alignment and movement efficiency by educating people to become aware of and modify their habitual habits. The Alexander Technique is still generally regarded for its usefulness in relieving stress and improving physical performance.

Moshe Feldenkrais (1904–1984): Moshe Feldenkrais, an Israeli physicist and judo master, developed the Feldenkrais Method following a crippling knee injury. Feldenkrais used his knowledge of physics, anatomy, and martial arts to create a method of gentle, mindful movements that improve self-awareness and functional movement. His technique teaches people new, healthier ways to move by emphasizing the nerve system's function in directing movement.

Ida Rolf (1896-1979) was an American scientist who invented Rolfing Structural Integration. Rolf felt that structural misalignments in the body were the root cause of chronic pain and dysfunction. Her approach combines deep tissue massage and movement teaching to help the body align with the gravitational field, creating balance and ease of movement. Rolfing is renowned for its tremendous effect on posture and structural alignment.

Thomas Hanna (1928–1990) was an American philosopher and movement educator who created the word "somatics" in the 1970s. He emphasized the body's experience from within and created Hanna Somatic Education, which focuses on retraining the nervous system to relieve chronic muscular tension and enhance movement patterns.

Hanna's work helped to popularize and integrate the notion of somatic education into modern practice.

Rudolf Laban (1879-1958): Rudolf Laban, a Hungarian dancer and thinker, developed Laban Movement Analysis, a system for studying and documenting human movement. Laban's framework has influenced dance, physical therapy, and somatic activities by giving a methodical approach to understanding and improving movement efficiency and expressiveness.

These pioneers paved the way for today's wide and extensive area of somatic activities. Their unique methods to movement and body awareness continue to influence and inspire future generations of practitioners, providing useful tools for improving physical and mental health. Understanding their contributions allows us to better comprehend the scope and complexity of somatic exercises, as well as their potential benefits.

Milestones in the Development of Somatic Practices

Over the past century, the field of somatic practices has changed thanks to the groundbreaking work of a number of significant personalities. The following are some significant turning points in the evolution of this revolutionary method of movement and body awareness:

The late 19th-century Alexander Technique: Actor Frederick Matthias Alexander created the Alexander Technique after experiencing vocal loss during a performance. He became aware that the way he was utilizing his body was affecting his ability to speak after closely examining himself. As a result, he developed a technique for retraining the mind-body link to enhance breathing, posture, and general movement patterns.

Early 20th-century Somatic Education's Emergence: Simultaneously, other noteworthy practitioners arose, such as Elsa Gindler, a German physical education instructor who used gentle, awareness-based exercises to help people rediscover their inner physiological wisdom. The discipline of somatic education, which emphasizes the first-hand experience of the live, sensed body, was thus founded.

The Mid-20th Century Founding of Somatic Therapy: Thomas Hanna, a philosopher and bodyworker, created Hanna Somatic Education, which focuses on releasing deeply ingrained reflexes and muscular tensions, building on the work of earlier pioneers. This method sought to relieve chronic pain and assist patients in taking back control of their movement patterns, much like other somatic therapies.

The Impact of Professional Dancers in the Late 20th Century: The development of somatic education was significantly influenced by the "body-mind thinking" of dance professionals as the area of somatic activities continued to evolve. Movement therapists and dancers have influenced the instruction and use of these approaches.

These and other significant events have influenced the diverse range of somatic therapies that are currently extensively employed to enhance mental, emotional, and physical health. By respecting the body's knowledge and fostering a more profound mind-body connection, somatic exercises enable people to move, feel, and live more effortlessly and vibrantly.

> "Somatic exercise isn't about achieving perfection, it's about embracing your body's unique journey. Start today and feel the difference with every mindful move."

CHAPTER 3

The Science Behind Somatic Exercises

Have you ever had a profound sense of calm wash over you after a mild yoga practice, or seen your persistent back pain improve after focusing on your posture? There is a reason behind that! Somatic exercises are more than just feeling good; they are supported by research, which explains the beneficial effects you notice.

Mind-Body Connection:

Think of your body and intellect as two sides of the same coin. Somatic exercises bridge this gap by altering your nervous system, which is the body's control center for movement and feeling. When we are stressed or anxious, our nervous system activates "fight-or-flight" mode, resulting in persistent muscular stiffness and discomfort. Somatic movements, which emphasize gentle exploration and awareness, indicate to your nervous system that it is safe to rest. This can reduce stress hormones and give you a sense of tranquility.

Reprogramming Movement Patterns:

Consider your everyday motions as well-worn routes built by your routines. Somatic exercises, which emphasize slow, controlled movements and self-observation, might help you discover these established habits. Consider slouching at your work without noticing it, or tense your shoulders when driving. Somatic awareness allows you to detect these tendencies and gently direct your body to more efficient and pain-free motions. Over time, these new, conscious motions become your new "paths," resulting in better posture, less discomfort, and a stronger sense of control over your body.

The Power of Neuroplasticity:

Our minds are more flexible than we realize! According to neuroplasticity science, our brains may develop new neural connections at any time during our lifetimes. Somatic exercises, which emphasize learning via movement and improving body awareness, increase the formation of new brain pathways associated to movement and feeling. This can result in enhanced motor control, more flexibility, and a stronger sensation of bodily connection.

So, the next time you feel at peace and relaxed after a Somatic exercise, remember: it's not your imagination! Science backs up the benefits of Somatic Exercises for your body and mind.

Understanding the Mind-Body Connection

Somatic exercises are based on the fundamental knowledge that our brains and bodies are intricately intertwined. This link between mind and body serves as the foundation for these transformational activities.

The mind-body connection is based on the idea that our ideas, emotions, and bodily experiences are all inextricably linked. Stress, worry, and trauma can all show as physical tension, pain, or discomfort in the body. In contrast, persistent physical behaviors, such as poor posture or muscular tension, can have an impact on our mental and emotional health.

Somatic exercises harness the power of the mind-body connection by urging you to focus your attention inward and become intensely aware of your body's sensations and motions. By developing this heightened body awareness, you will be able to detect the subtle ways in which your ideas and feelings manifest physically. This helps you to make mindful modifications and break free from any unhelpful patterns that may be causing discomfort or malfunction.

Somatic exercises will teach you how to listen to your body's knowledge and respond with love and care. As you become more aware of your physical self's subtle signals, you will discover that you are better able to handle stress, control your emotions, and maintain an overall feeling of well-being. Imagine the relaxation you'll experience as chronic tension and discomfort melt away, leaving your body with a renewed feeling of ease and fluidity. This is the strength of the mind-body connection: it is about building a profound, harmonious link between your ideas, feelings, and bodily experience, rather than just physical health.

As you continue to learn about somatic exercises, keep in mind that you are embarking on a profound path of self-discovery and empowerment. Honoring the delicate dance between your mind and body opens up a world of healing, development, and transformation.

Research and Evidence

Somatic exercises may appear novel, but scientific study has produced a growing amount of data supporting their efficacy. While somatic techniques vary, the fundamental concepts of mindful movement and body awareness show promise in a variety of contexts. Let's look at some major findings:

- ❖ **Pain Relief and Management:** Chronic pain has a tremendous influence on our lives. According to studies, somatic exercises such as the Feldenkrais Method may help manage chronic pain issues such as back pain, neck pain, and headaches. These exercises assist people in identifying and releasing stress patterns that cause pain, so facilitating healing and preventing future issues.

- ❖ **Improved mobility and flexibility.** Feeling stiff and inflexible? Somatic exercise can assist! According to studies, activities such as the Alexander Technique can help increase flexibility and range of motion. This can lead to improved performance in daily activities, such as reaching for a high shelf or bending down to tie your shoes with ease.

- ❖ **Stress Reduction and Mental Wellbeing:** The relationship between the mind and the body is reciprocal. Somatic exercises, which emphasize breathwork and gentle movement, can be an effective therapy for stress and anxiety management. According to research, somatic activities can reduce stress hormones while also promoting relaxation and well-being.

- **Enhanced body awareness:** Imagine being fully present in your own body. Somatic exercises help you become more conscious of your body's sensations. According to research, increased awareness can improve proprioception, or your body's sense of position and movement in space. This can help in hobbies like dance, athletics, and even daily duties like walking and sitting.
- **Important to Remember:** While the research is promising, the discipline of Somatic Research is still developing. Studies sometimes include small groups of individuals, and additional study is required to fully comprehend the long-term impact of Somatic practices on diverse illnesses.
- **Beyond the Numbers: Personal Experience Matters.** The genuine power of Somatic Exercises is based not only on scientific proof but also on personal experience. Many people who include somatic techniques in their daily lives report feeling better, having better posture, and experiencing less discomfort. Finally, the rewards you receive are what counts most.

The Neuroscience of Movement and Awareness

The core of somatic exercises is the complex interconnection between movement, consciousness, and the brain. By developing a more profound comprehension of the relationship between the mind and body, you may access the whole capabilities of these activities that bring about significant changes. The key to understanding the neurology of somatic workouts resides in the idea of proprioception - the body's ability to detect its location, motions, and activities. By participating in somatic activities, you actively strengthen your inherent self-awareness, enabling you to discern minute alterations and feelings inside your body.

The enhanced sense of body position and movement, known as heightened proprioception, is supported by the motor cortex. The motor cortex is a brain area situated beneath the frontal lobe and is responsible for controlling voluntary motions. The motor cortex transmits neural signals via the brain stem, spinal cord, and neural network to the targeted muscles, inducing them to contract.

Nevertheless, the correlation between movement and consciousness is more intricate than previously believed. Mounting evidence indicates that the awareness of purpose does not arise suddenly, but rather develops gradually over time. The early brain indicators of choice outcomes are not subconscious, but instead, they indicate the conscious appraisal stages of goals that are still in progress and hence not yet reported. By comprehending the neuroscientific principles behind movement and consciousness, one can acquire the ability to utilize the potential of the mind-body correlation. Through frequent practice, you'll acquire a deeper knowledge of your body's feelings and emotions, helping you to relieve chronic tension, increase flexibility, and boost general well-being.

To fully reap the advantages of somatic exercises, it is crucial to understand the dynamic relationship between physical movement, conscious awareness, and the brain. By tapping into this fundamental connection, you may start on a journey of self-discovery and empowerment, altering the way you move, feel, and live.

Practical Application

As a novice discovering the realm of somatic exercises, you may be wondering: how can I apply these ideas and practices to my daily life? The beauty of somatic exercises resides in their variety and accessibility, allowing you to smoothly integrate them into your routine and receive the advantages.

Incorporating Somatic Exercises into Your Morning Routine

Starting your day with somatic exercises may be a great way to set the tone for the rest of your day. Begin by spending a few seconds to listen into your body, recognizing any areas of tension or discomfort. Gently go through some easy stretches or body scans, allowing your awareness to lead the motions. This might help you feel more grounded, centered, and ready to take on the day ahead.

Practicing Somatic Awareness During Daily Activities

Somatic exercises aren't restricted to specific practice periods. You may use the ideas of body awareness and mindful movement for different elements of your everyday life, such as home tasks, strolling, or even sitting at your computer. As you go about your chores, pay attention to how your body feels and make minor modifications to maintain your posture and alignment.

Utilizing Somatic Strategies for Stress Management

When life gets stressful, somatic exercises may be a useful tool for stress release and emotional management. Practices like breathwork, grounding exercises, and gentle movement can help quiet the nervous system and offer a sense of embodied safety. By listening to your physical feelings, you may learn to detect and release stress before it worsens.

Exploring Somatic Approaches to Movement and Exercise

Whether you're an avid athlete or someone who enjoys more mild kinds of movement, somatic exercises can enrich your whole physical experience. By focusing on the quality of your movements rather than the number, you may increase your flexibility, balance, and coordination while lowering the chance of injury.

As you continue to explore the realm of somatic exercises, remember to approach your practice with patience, curiosity, and self-compassion. Everybody is unique, and what works for one person may not work for another. Trust your intuition, listen to your body's cues, and make modifications as required. With consistent practice, you'll uncover the transforming potential of somatic exercises, helping you to move, feel, and live with increased ease and energy.

"Beyond the poses, beyond the pain. Somatic Exercise for Beginners is your path to a deeper connection with yourself, one gentle movement at a time."

CHAPTER 4

Basic Somatic Exercises

If you're interested in somatic stretching, here are five beginner-friendly techniques to explore. Warren suggests practicing each for around five minutes and doing it every day.

1. Standing Awareness.

Warren advocates merely standing and becoming aware of various muscles in your body before proceeding with any additional somatic stretches.

- Stand up straight with your feet planted. Take note of how they grasp the floor.
- Try contracting and relaxing your foot muscles.
- Take deep breaths and notice how your abdominal muscles stretch and contract, as well as how it feels.
- Finally, examine your body from top to bottom, and notice how each muscle feels. Locate any points of strain.

2. Hang your head.

Keator shows how this practice might help relieve stress in our necks.

- Stand upright with your feet firmly planted on the ground.
- Slowly hang your head, allowing it to fall as far as it can safely go.

- Consider how the muscles in your neck feel and how the movement has affected neighboring muscles, joints, and tissues, such as your shoulders and upper back.
- Identify a tight location, such as the back of your neck, and really explore how it feels.
- Notice how it feels to relax into the stretch and attempt to relieve some of the tension.

3. Arch and Flatten

If you have back discomfort, Warren advises the arch and flatten technique, which helps you to relax and then restore control of the muscles in your lower back and abdomen. It is a slow movement performed while lying on the floor.

- Position your feet level on the floor, hip-distance apart, and knees bent.
- Take a deep breath and pay attention to how the muscles in your lower back and abdominals move.
- Gently arch your back, pulling your belly up and squeezing your glutes and feet into the floor.
- Stay thus for as long as you feel comfortable, then gradually lower your back and flatten it on the floor.
- Repeat the action gently, assessing the muscles in your torso for any tension and attempting to release it.

4. Iliopsoas Exercise.

The iliopsoas is the muscle group that connects your spine to your legs, and it is the source of much strain for many of us. According to Warren, this exercise increases awareness of these and neighboring muscles, allowing you to release tension more effectively.

- ❖ Lie on your back, knees bent, and feet flat on the floor.
- ❖ Put your right hand behind your head.
- ❖ Lift your head gently while simultaneously lifting your right leg, keeping it bent and roughly 6 inches off the floor. (This should resemble a crunch on one side of your body.)
- ❖ Scan the muscles in your lower back, hips, and legs for tightness and note how they feel.
- ❖ Gently lower your leg and head.
- ❖ Repeat, but this time straighten your leg slightly as you rise.
- ❖ Repeat these motions slowly and softly several times, then repeat on the opposite side.

5. Carpal Tunnel Exercise

If you spend a lot of time typing on a computer or other device, Warren suggests that this exercise might help relieve stress in your waist, shoulders, chest, hands, and wrists.

- ❖ Lie on your left side, knees bent at a 90-degree angle in front of you, head resting on your left arm (which can be bent or straight).
- ❖ Place your right hand on the floor, upper arm resting on your torso, elbow bent at approximately a 90-degree angle.

- Move your right arm up and around your head, keeping your right hand near your left ear and your elbow pointing straight up.
- Gently guide your head to the ceiling with your hand, contracting the right side of your waist. (This resembles a side crunch.) Take note of how those muscles flex.
- When you're ready, release and softly lower your head back down. Repeat once.
- Roll softly onto your back, right elbow toward the ceiling, and right arm behind your head.
- Bring your left arm to the side.
- Crunch your right arm, shoulder, and head up and to the left side of your body.
- Release and slowly drop your head and shoulders. Repeat these actions on the opposite side.

Preparing for Practice

Starting your somatic exercise adventure requires the proper mentality and preparation. This is more than simply physical motions; it is about developing a profound, embodied awareness that may affect all aspects of your life. First and foremost, remember to be patient and loving towards yourself. Somatic exercises are about connecting with your body's particular knowledge rather than striving for perfection. There is no one-size-fits-all strategy, so allow your body to lead you to the techniques that work best for you.

When you're ready to start, choose a quiet, comfortable place where you can move freely and without distractions. This may be your living room, a quiet part of your lawn, or even a designated meditation space. Dim the lights, put on some calming music, and allow yourself to relax in the present now.

As you settle in, take a few deep breaths and check your body for any points of tension or discomfort. Gently draw your attention to these areas, acknowledging them without judgment. Imagine embracing them in a loving, calming hug, letting the tension gently melt away.

Now focus on your breathing. Feel the air going in and out, taking note of the natural rhythm and flow. Allow your breath to serve as an anchor, bringing you back to the present moment and assisting you in letting go of any lingering anxieties or distractions.

Finally, have a clear aim for your practice. This might be as simple as wanting to feel more connected to your body or setting a particular goal, such as improving your posture or eliminating back discomfort. Allow this desire to permeate and direct your motions while you explore. Remember that the key to a successful somatic practice is to approach it with an open heart and an inquisitive mind. Embrace the journey, believe in your body's wisdom, and be patient with yourself as you discover the transforming potential of these exercises. With each practice, you'll strengthen your connection with yourself and achieve new levels of physical, mental, and emotional well-being.

Essential Warm-Up Exercises

Before beginning your somatic exercises, be sure to warm up your body gently. This will improve blood flow, lower the chance of injury, and pave the way for a more successful and pleasurable practice. Here are some basic warm-up activities to get you started:

Leg Swings.

- ❖ Stand shoulder-width apart, hands on hips. Swing your legs back and forth, with your knees slightly bent. Feel a mild stretch in your hamstrings and glutes. As you swing, concentrate on the feelings in your legs and the rhythm of your breathing.

Arm Circles

- ❖ Stand shoulder-width apart, arms outstretched to the sides. Make tiny circles with your arms while keeping your shoulders relaxed and elbows straight. Feel a mild stretch in your shoulders and rotation in your upper back. As you circle, concentrate on the feelings in your arms and the fluid movement of your joints.

Neck Rolls

- ❖ Stand with feet shoulder-width apart and hands on hips. Slowly tilt your head to one side, placing your ear near your shoulder. Hold for a bit, then return to the middle. Repeat on the opposite side. Feel the mild stretch in your neck and the relief from tension in your shoulders.

Shoulder Roll

- ❖ To perform shoulder rolls, stand with hands on hips and feet shoulder-width apart. Slowly move your shoulders forward and backward, experiencing a mild stretch in your upper back and the relief of tension in your neck. Repeat numerous times, concentrating on the feelings in your shoulders and the fluid movement of your joints.
- ❖ Warm up by breathing deeply and focusing on your body's feelings. Allow yourself to fully engage in the motions, releasing any tension or discomfort. Preparing your body with these crucial warm-up exercises will allow you to delve into your somatic practice with confidence and ease.

Beginner-Friendly Somatic Movements

As a beginner exploring the world of somatic exercises, you may be wondering where to start. The beauty of these practices is that they can be tailored to all levels, allowing you to gradually build your awareness and confidence. Let's dive into some beginner-friendly somatic movements that can help you cultivate a deeper mind-body connection.

Rocking and Rolling

- ✤ Imagine yourself lying comfortably on your back, knees bent, and feet flat on the floor. Gently rock your knees from side to side, feeling the gentle sway of your spine. As you rock, pay attention to the sensations in your body and the rhythm of your breath. This simple movement can help release tension in your back and hips, while also promoting a sense of calm and grounding.

Pelvic Tilts

- Remain on your back, with your knees bent and feet flat on the floor. Slowly tilt your pelvis forward, feeling the gentle arch in your lower back. Then, tilt your pelvis back, allowing your lower back to flatten against the floor. Repeat this movement, focusing on the subtle shifts in your body and the connection between your mind and your core.

Shoulder Circles

- Stand with your feet shoulder-width apart, arms hanging loosely at your sides. Slowly begin to circle your shoulders, first forward and then backward. As you move, pay attention to the sensations in your upper back and shoulders, allowing the movement to be smooth and effortless. This exercise can help release tension in your neck and shoulders, while also improving your overall posture.

Ankle Rolls

- Sit or stand with your feet hip-width apart. Slowly begin to circle your ankles, first in one direction and then the other. Feel the gentle stretch and rotation in your ankles, and notice how this simple movement can have a calming effect on your body and mind.

As you explore these beginner-friendly somatic movements, remember to approach them with patience, curiosity, and self-compassion. There's no right or wrong way to do them - the key is to tune in to your body's signals and move in a way that feels good and nourishing for you. With regular practice, you'll begin to unlock the transformative power of somatic exercises, empowering you to move, feel, and live with greater ease and vitality.

> "Don't be intimidated, be inspired. Somatic Exercise welcomes everyone, regardless of age or fitness level. Start your journey today!"

CHAPTER 5

Targeting Common Problem Areas.

As a beginner exploring the realm of somatic exercises, you may be wondering how these practices might help with some of the most prevalent physical difficulties. The beauty of somatic exercises is their ability to address particular problem regions while providing long-term comfort.

Relieving back pain

Do you ever feel rushed, busy, or overwhelmed? If you're like me, it might give you the feeling of always being on the go, with a mindset that goes something like "I'll be able to relax once I get (fill in the blank) done." Your muscles react to every idea and feeling that you experience. Isn't it amazing? It helps me understand how the mind and body are one. It also explains why, if you have this sensation of activity for a long time, you may develop persistent lower back discomfort or stiffness even when you are not stressed. Why is this happening?

Simply explained, your brain regulates your muscles.

So, every time the alarm goes off, you hurry to catch the bus, or you think, "I have a million things to do today," your back muscles contract to assist you move ahead and do all of your tasks.

Now, this isn't a negative thing in and of itself, and it can also be a joyful response - a "yes" to life; it only becomes a problem when it becomes a habitual way of living your life. Your muscles can learn to stay "on" even when not needed, similar to how learning to ride a bicycle or play the piano becomes natural and requires no conscious effort. This explains why, even when you desire to relax, your muscles might stay stiff and painful.

Your brain has "forgotten" that your muscles are half contracted. It's called Sensory-Motor Amnesia (SMA), It sounds alarming, but having SMA to some level is fairly typical - and not unexpectedly, considering the fast-paced nature of our culture and the amount of stimulation in our surroundings, it frequently leads to tight back muscles, which can result in lower back discomfort over time. You can teach your brain to relax tight, stiff, and painful muscles. It is possible to release and relax your muscles, relieving stiffness and soreness. The secret is a strange-sounding procedure known as pandiculation, which you can only do on yourself. Pandiculation is a natural activity for all vertebrate creatures, with research indicating that animals pandiculate 42 times every day. **Pandiculation is nature's technique to wake up the brain.**

A pandiculation consists of three components:

1. You contract a muscle tighter than it currently is (this wakes up the brain and allows it to begin to detect the constricted muscle).

2. You gradually release and extend the muscle (the brain relearns how to release and relax the muscle to its normal length).
3. You totally relax at the conclusion (so that the brain can detect how a relaxed muscle feels).

Here is a simple Somatic Exercise to Release the Lower Back.

Practicing this action every day to maintain my back muscles relaxed and under voluntary control of my brain. Even if you don't already have lower back discomfort, this activity is excellent for avoiding it.

Step 1: Listen to your body.

Begin by reclining comfortably on your back, legs bent, and feet flat on the ground. Take a few deep breaths, then begin scanning your body, focusing particularly on your back. Take note of any regions of tension or discomfort, as well as the location of your pain.

Step 2: Arch and flatten.

Gently arch your lower back, feeling the soft curvature in your spine. Hold for a bit, then gradually release and let your back flatten to the floor. Repeat this action while paying attention to your body feelings and breathing pattern. This exercise can assist to relieve stress in the back muscles and enhance spinal mobility.

Step 3: Pelvic tilts.

Continue to lie on your back with your knees bent and feet flat on the floor. Slowly tilt your pelvis forward to feel the soft arch in your lower back. Then, tilt your pelvis back and let your lower back flatten on the floor. Repeat this action, focusing on the tiny changes in your body and the link between your mind and your core.

Step 4: Integrate Awareness.

As you progress through these exercises, strive to develop a stronger feeling of bodily awareness. Observe how your breath changes, how your muscles react, and how your overall sensation of ease and comfort evolves. This increased awareness is the key to realizing the transforming potential of somatic exercises. Note, that the route to relief from back pain is unique to each individual, and what works for one person may not for another. Approach your practice with patience, self-compassion, and an eagerness to experiment. With consistent somatic exercise, you might start to notice a significant reduction in back discomfort and a revitalized sensation of mobility in your body.

Improving posture

Improving your posture may be a transforming experience when you are new to somatic exercises. By developing a stronger mind-body connection, you may reduce chronic stress and retrain your nervous system to promote a healthier, more aligned posture. Let's go over a step-by-step instruction to help you get started.

Step 1: Listen to your body.

Start by standing tall with your feet shoulder-width apart. Take a few deep breaths and begin scanning your body, paying close attention to your spine, shoulders, and head. Take notice of any tightness or pain in your body.

Step 2: Shoulder rolls.

Slowly move your shoulders forward and backward, experiencing a mild stretch in your upper back and the relief of tension in your neck. As you move, concentrate on your body's feelings and the smooth, fluid action of your shoulders. This practice can assist in relieving chronic tension and improve your overall posture.

Step 3: Neck Rolls.

Tilt your head to one side and bring your ear near your shoulder. Hold for a moment before gently returning to the center. Repeat on the opposite side, experiencing the gradual stretch in your neck and the relief of tension in your shoulders. This simple exercise can reduce neck discomfort and improve head alignment.

Step 4: Pelvic tilts.

Stand shoulder-width apart, hands on hips. Slowly tilt your pelvis forward to feel the soft arch in your lower back. Then, tilt your pelvis back and let your lower back flatten on the floor. Repeat this exercise, focusing on the small changes in your body and the link between your core and spine.

Step 5: Integrate Awareness.

As you progress through these exercises, strive to develop a stronger feeling of bodily awareness. Observe how your breath changes, how your muscles react, and how your overall sensation of ease and comfort evolves. This increased awareness is the key to realizing the transforming potential of somatic exercises.

Remember that changing your posture is a process, not a destination. Approach your practice with patience, self-compassion, and an eagerness to experiment. With frequent somatic exercise, you can start to notice a significant improvement in your physical, mental, and emotional well-being, allowing you to move, feel, and live more freely and vitally.

Key benefits of practicing somatic exercises for posture

Here are the main advantages of doing somatic exercises to improve posture:

Reduces chronic muscle tension.

Somatic activities relieve deep-seated muscle stress, which contributes to bad posture. Somatic techniques help the muscles release chronic contraction patterns by fostering a heightened awareness of the body and employing gentle movements.

Re-trains proprioception.

Proprioception refers to the body's capacity to detect its location and motions. Poor posture becomes habitual when the proprioceptive and vestibular systems adjust to a slouched or misaligned stance. Somatic techniques retrain proprioception by teaching the body how proper posture feels inside.

Improves Flexibility and Mobility

Somatic stretches, as opposed to dynamic stretching, include holding postures that improve joint flexibility and range of motion. This greater flexibility promotes good posture and lowers the chance of injury.

Enhances body awareness.

Somatic activities promote a stronger mind-body connection and an understanding of how emotions affect posture. Tuning into bodily sensations allows you to notice and release tension before it causes poor alignment.

Provides objective feedback.

Mirrors or photographs give an impartial, third-person perspective of your stance. This helps you to match what you're feeling inside with how your posture appears. The mirror provides rapid feedback on right and faulty alignment.

Reduces stress and anxiety.

Somatic techniques such as breathwork and meditation assist to soothe the nervous system and reduce emotions of tension and anxiety. As these unpleasant emotions frequently lead to bad posture, eliminating them promotes better alignment.

Somatic activities improve posture holistically by releasing chronic muscular tension, retraining proprioception, and increasing body awareness. With frequent practice and repetition, these exercises can result in long-term posture modifications as well as reduced pain or discomfort.

How emotions influence our posture and how somatic exercises can help.

Here's an overview of how emotions affect posture and how somatic exercises might help:

How Emotions Influence Posture.

- ✓ Emotions are represented through our body posture and muscular tone. A slumped, closed-off posture might be indicative of dread, anxiety, or low self-esteem.
- ✓ In contrast, an upright, open stance can indicate confidence, optimism, and a sense of security.
- ✓ Stress and unpleasant emotions can cause muscular tension and bad posture, therefore the autonomic nervous system plays an important role.
- ✓ Emotions and posture interact in a bidirectional manner; our posture may impact how we feel emotionally.

How Do Somatic Exercises Help?

- ✓ Somatic exercises use gentle, attentive movements to increase body awareness and relieve chronic muscular tension.
- ✓ Somatic techniques, which focus on bodily sensations and movement patterns, can help retrain the nervous system and break bad posture habits.
- ✓ Specific somatic exercises, such as shoulder rolls, neck rolls, and pelvic tilts, can help to relieve stress and improve overall posture.
- ✓ The mind-body link is essential since somatic exercises teach you to watch how emotions emerge physically and make conscious adjustments.
- ✓ Regular somatic practice can result in long-term gains in posture, flexibility, and emotional stability.

The idea is to view posture as a whole, embodied experience rather than merely an exterior look. Somatic exercises allow you to adopt an active, aware approach to improving your posture and general well-being.

Enhancing flexibility

As a novice exploring the realm of somatic exercises, you may want to enhance your flexibility and range of motion. Unlike standard stretching regimens, which can feel forced or painful, somatic activities provide a softer, more natural way to build flexibility. Let's go over a step-by-step instruction to help you get started.

Step 1: Listen to your body.

❖ Begin by choosing a comfortable sitting or laying posture. Take a few deep breaths and begin scanning your body, paying close attention to any regions that seem tight or constricted. Pay attention to the feelings in your muscles and joints, and make a mental note of where you feel the most tightness. This moment of self-awareness is critical because it allows you to customize the workouts to your own requirements.

Step 2: Leg Swings.

❖ Begin gently swinging your legs back and forth while keeping your knees slightly bent. As you move, concentrate on the feelings in your hamstrings and glutes, enabling the action to be fluid and effortless. Imagine your muscles loosening and releasing with each swing as if you were melting away any remaining tension. This easy exercise might help you improve hip and lower-body mobility.

Step 3: Ankle Rolls.

❖ Direct your focus to your feet and ankles. Begin slowly circling your ankles, first in one direction, then the other. Feel the mild stretch and rotation in your joints, and observe how this simple action may soothe both your body and mind. Targeting the ankles improves general flexibility and balance.

As you get more familiar with these fundamental somatic exercises, accept your body's guidance and experiment with various motions that feel nourishing and helpful. Remember, the objective is to approach your practice with patience, self-compassion, and an openness to your body's cues. With consistent practice, you will notice a significant improvement in your flexibility, as well as a greater feeling of embodied awareness and overall well-being.

Reducing tension in the neck and shoulders

- When you roll your neck to relieve stress after staring at your phone for too long, you are automatically doing somatic stretching. It is your body's way of relieving aching, overworked muscles.
- Stress, traumas, and repetitive activity can all cause muscles to become chronically stiff over time. This might have a detrimental influence on your emotions and movements.
- "The goal of somatic stretching is to turn inward, become aware of where you're holding tension, and use your breath and gentle movement to release built-up stress in your body," explains CentraState health coach and mind-body specialist Beth Ando-Brenman, MPT. "The breath powers the mind-body connection - it's the key to relieving tension and feeling centered and calm."
- Somatic exercises help release stress and tension from your muscles and mind.

Do you want to experience the relaxing effects of somatic stretching? Begin with these basic exercises to reduce stress in your neck, shoulders, and back. To help you ground yourself and strengthen your mind-body connection, do each exercise in a comfortable, sitting position—on a chair or cross-legged on the floor, spine extended. Perform each exercise for one to two minutes, moving thoughtfully from one to the next. Somatic stretches may be done at any time, but they are especially useful at the beginning and end of the day.

Relieving Neck Stress

Step 1: Lower your chin to your chest, gently into the stretch with your breath.

Step 2: Return your chin to its starting position and gradually lower your right ear to your right shoulder, just until you feel a mild tug. Do the same thing on the opposing side.

Step 3: Repeat the process from the start for one to two minutes.

Releasing Shoulder Tension

Step 1: Keep the back of your neck long and your shoulders low.

Step 2: Inhale and roll your shoulders back and down on the exhale, leaving space between your ears and the tops of your shoulders.

Step 3: Reverse the movement. Inhale and lift your shoulders back, up to your ears, then down.

Step 4: Repeat this several times in both directions, using a smooth, rolling motion.

Open Up the Chest and Upper Back

Step 1: Put your hands on your knees, inhale, and bring your chest up. Your shoulders will instinctively draw back. If you can, raise your chin slightly to enable the stretch to reach the front of your neck. (If your lower back is arching too much, thrust your pelvis forward slightly.)

Step 2: When you feel a great stretch across your chest, exhale, lower your chin to your chest, and round your shoulders and upper back inward as if you were making the top of a "O" with your upper body. This will stretch and relieve your upper back.

Step 3: Repeat the sequence, moving smoothly from one to the other.

Releasing Spinal and Lower Back Tension

Step 1: Sit with your feet firmly planted on the ground or cross-legged on the floor. Place your left palm on the outside of your right knee and your right palm or fingertips behind you on the seat or floor. Your right arm should be a few inches out from your body and exactly behind your right shoulder, straight but not locked—like a kickstand for your body. If you're seated in a chair, move up to the front edge to allow room for your back arm.

Step 2: Inhale, stretch your spine, then exhale and slowly rotate to the right, moving your head in the same direction. Press your left palm on the outside of your right knee to generate some traction. It should feel like you are gently wringing out your spine. Twist until it feels right for you.

Step 3: Breathe into it and repeat on the opposite side.

Completing these four somatic stretches will help you feel relaxed and tension-free—both physically and mentally.

Somatic strategies for stress reduction

We've all experienced clammy hands, racing hearts, and overpowering dread and fear. Anxiety is a common part of life. In fact, feeling nervous might be beneficial in some situations. It keeps you awake, keeps you secure, and encourages you to improve your behavior. But what if this becomes a never-ending cycle? When left unchecked, it has the potential to completely dominate your life. Fortunately, somatic skills can help you handle stress and anxiety more successfully.

4. Unleash Your Body's Wisdom Through Movement.

The body is one of our most powerful and expressive vehicles. To access its knowledge, we must engage in movement.

When we exercise, our bodies naturally release endorphins, which act as mood boosters and stress relievers. They assist in changing our emotional state from negative to positive and give us a sense of tranquility.

This might take any form—yoga, dancing, running, hiking—whatever appeals to you. The idea is to keep the exercise light and entertaining, not overwhelming or difficult.

If you're having trouble motivating yourself, consider taking a fitness class or planning a trek with family and friends. Developing camaraderie may be a tremendous source of inspiration!

In addition to movement-based activities, you can do grounding techniques such as strolling barefoot on grass and absorbing the sights, sounds, and scents around you. These simple tasks help us become more present and attentive of our surroundings.

5. Setting a Routine for Self-Care

Creating a self-care regimen might seem like a difficult job, especially when suffering from worry and stress.

But you're making time to care for the most important person in your life: yourself.

Even five minutes each day may make a major difference, laying the groundwork for long-term change and putting you in control of your mental health and well-being. It also helps you restore your relationship with your inner child, who is frequently ignored and pushed aside while we are preoccupied with our everyday chores.

Here are some excellent options to try:

- Take a vacation from social media and your smart gadgets.
- Read a book.
- Spend time outside in nature.
- Take a warm bubble bath in the evenings after work.
- Light some candles or incense to create a relaxing mood.

Applying awareness to household chores

You may be wondering how to incorporate these revolutionary techniques into your daily life. One of the most appealing aspects of somatic exercises is their ability to be smoothly integrated into even the most monotonous of duties, such as domestic chores. As you fold the clothes, imagine paying full attention to your body's feelings. Feel the fabric's weight in your hands and the delicate stretch as you smooth each piece. Take note of the rhythm of your breath and the small adjustments in your posture as you move. A single act of attention may turn a tiresome task into a peaceful experience.

Imagine yourself doing the dishes, warm water pouring over your hands. As you scrub and rinse, take note of the temperature of the water, the texture of the sponge, and the movement of your arms. Allow yourself to totally engage in the current moment rather than allowing your attention stray to the never-ending to-do list. Even something as simple as sweeping the floor might provide a chance to develop somatic awareness. Feel the connection between your feet and the ground, and allow your body to sway gently while you move the broom back and forth. Observe the minute changes in your weight and balance, as well as how your muscles adapt to the work at hand.

The benefit of integrating somatic awareness to domestic duties is that it requires no more time or effort. Simply focus your attention within, tune into your body's feelings, and allow the motions to emerge with presence and intention. As you negotiate your regular duties with this increased awareness, you may notice a significant change in your experience. The stress and boredom of tasks can fade away, leaving behind a sense of serenity, grounding, and even a renewed appreciation for the modest joys of home life.

So, the next time you're elbow-deep in dishes or folding another load of clothes, remember to take a break, breathe, and reconnect with your body's knowledge. The actual power of somatic exercises can be experienced in these seemingly ordinary times.

Somatic principles for walking and running

As someone new discovering the realm of somatic exercises, you may be astonished to realize that even the most fundamental activities, such as walking and running, may be modified via a stronger mind-body connection. By integrating somatic practice concepts into your daily tasks, you may achieve a new level of ease, efficiency, and total well-being.

Grounding and Stability

Walking and running require a solid foundation. Begin by focusing on your connection to the ground and feeling your body's weight evenly distributed through your feet. Imagine your feet as roots that attach you to the ground and provide a secure foundation for your motions. This sensation of grounding can help you feel more focused and in control, lowering your risk of injury and increasing your sense of comfort.

Proprioceptive Awareness.

Proprioception refers to the body's capacity to detect its own location and motions in space. By developing a better understanding of your body's location and how your limbs move, you may make tiny changes to your gait and running form, increasing efficiency and decreasing strain on your joints and muscles.

Breath and rhythm.

The rhythm of your breathing may have a significant influence on how you move. As you walk or run, pay attention to the natural flow of your inhalations and exhalations, allowing your body to move in tandem with this internal rhythm. This can help you save energy, decrease stress, and improve your overall sense of well-being.

Mindful Presence

Rather than allowing your thoughts to stray to the never-ending to-do list or the unpleasantness of the task, practice mindful presence. Pay attention to the feelings in your body, the sound of your footsteps, and the environment around you. This increased awareness may elevate even the most ordinary chores into contemplative experiences, filling your movement with joy and vibrancy.

Incorporating these somatic concepts into your walking and running routines, will not only enhance the physical elements of these exercises but also gain a deeper connection to your body and the world around you. Accept the trip and appreciate the transforming effects of movement with somatic awareness.

Mindful sitting and standing

These simple yet effective exercises can help you develop a stronger mind-body connection, decrease stress, and boost your general well-being.

Mindful Sitting.

Step one: Find a comfortable position.

Begin by sitting comfortably, back straight, feet flat on the floor. Take a few deep breaths and let your body relax into the present moment.

Step Two: Body Scan

Slowly scan your body, beginning at your toes and progressing to your head. Take notice of any places of tension or discomfort, and consider how each part of your body feels.

Step 3: Breathing Awareness

Focus your attention on your breath. Feel the air going in and out of your nose, and observe how your body reacts to each inhale and expiration.

Step 4: Posture adjustment.

Gently alter your posture to keep your back straight and your shoulders relaxed. Imagine your body as a tree, firmly planted in the earth, with your head lifted high and your chest open.

Mindful Standing

Step 1: Grounding.

Stand shoulder-width apart and feel your body's weight equally distributed through your feet. Imagine your feet as roots that anchor you to the ground.

Step 2: Body Awareness.

Scan your body from head to toe, noting any points of tension or discomfort. Concentrate on the feelings in your feet, legs, and torso, and allow your body to return to its natural position.

Step 3: Breath and Movement.

Observe how your body moves with each inhale and expiration. Feel your chest gently rising and falling, as well as the movement of your diaphragm.

Step 4: Posture adjustment.

Gently alter your posture to keep your back straight and your shoulders relaxed. Imagine your body as a tower, powerful and stable, with your head lifted high and your chest wide.

Benefits of Mindful Sitting and Standing

- **Reduced tension:** By concentrating on your breath and body, you may reduce tension and anxiety, encouraging a state of peace and relaxation.
- **Improved Posture**: Regular practice can help you maintain excellent posture, lower your risk of back problems, and improve your overall physical health.
- **Enhanced Body Awareness**: Mindful sitting and standing can help you get a better knowledge of your body's feelings and motions, increasing your sense of embodiment.
- **Increased Mindfulness**: These exercises can help you build mindfulness in your daily activities, helping you to be more present and focused in all parts of your life.

Remember, the key to these exercises is to approach them with patience, self-compassion, and an eagerness to learn. By adopting attentive sitting and standing into your daily routine, you may achieve a new level of comfort, balance, and well-being.

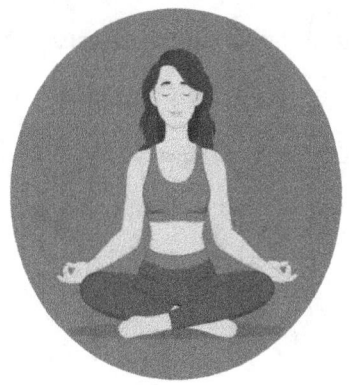

CHAPTER 6

Overcoming Common Challenges

As a novice exploring the realm of bodily workouts, you may face frequent obstacles that impede your growth. However, by knowing these obstacles and adopting the proper mentality, you may overcome them and achieve your objectives. Here are some suggestions to assist you in overcoming typical obstacles:

1. Lack of consistency.

Somatic exercises require consistency to obtain their full advantages. Begin by making a timetable and sticking to it. Find the optimum time for you and make it a non-negotiable component of your daily schedule. Remember that even tiny initiatives can result in considerable growth over time.

2. Physical discomfort.

Physical pain is a typical issue, particularly when beginning out. Listen to your body and make adjustments to your workouts as needed. If something causes discomfort, consider adjusting the movement or moving to a different activity. Remember, the purpose is to feel good, not to endure pain.

3. Mental Blocks.

Fear of failing or overwhelming emotions might cause mental barriers. Recognize these emotions and remind yourself that everyone begins somewhere. Concentrate on the present moment and the progress you're making rather than the ultimate objective. Celebrate minor accomplishments and keep motivated.

4. Lack of progress.

It's normal to get upset when development appears slow. Instead of becoming disappointed, use this as a chance to analyze and adapt your strategy. Consider consulting a professional somatic practitioner or trying out different exercises to find what works best for you.

5. Self-doubt

Self-doubt might set in when you don't see instant results. Remember, somatic exercises are a journey, not a destination. Focus on the process rather than the end. Practice self-compassion and recognize that everyone learns at their own rate.

6. Time constraints.

Making time for somatic exercises might be difficult, especially with a hectic schedule. Begin by introducing small sessions into your regular schedule. As you gain confidence in the exercises, gradually increase the time.

7. Lack of support

A supportive community may mean all the difference. Join online forums or search for local groups that share your interests. Share your experience and learn from others. This can help keep you motivated and accountable.

8. Fear of the unknown.

Fear of the unknown may be overwhelming. Approach each new activity with interest and eagerness to learn. Concentrate on the sensations in your body and the moves you are performing. This might help you feel more in control and less anxious.

Addressing these typical issues allows you to overcome hurdles and make considerable progress on your somatic exercise journey. Remember to be patient, kind, and open-minded. With consistent practice and a good attitude, you may experience the transforming advantages of somatic exercises and develop a stronger mind-body connection.

Addressing Common Beginner Mistakes

It is expected to experience a few setbacks along the way. However, by being aware of these typical mistakes and approaching them with patience and self-compassion, you may avoid them and fully realize the transformational impact of these practices.

Trying too hard.

One of the most typical mistakes made by novices is putting too much effort into somatic exercises. Remember, the goal of these activities is to cultivate a gentle, attentive awareness of your body rather than pushing yourself to the point of discomfort. Slow down, breathe deeply, and let the movements happen naturally.

Rushing through the exercises.

Somatic exercises are about the process, not the outcome. Resist the impulse to speed through the exercises; instead, take your time to appreciate each sensation and shift in your body truly. This cautious, methodical approach is essential for retraining your neural system and establishing long-term improvement.

Comparing Yourself with Others

It's easy to fall into the trap of comparing your own development to that of others. Remember that everyone's path is unique. Instead of stressing about how you compare to your classmates, focus on your own experiences and appreciate minor achievements.

Neglecting the Mind-Body Connection.

Somatic exercises are more than simply physical motions; they also aim to increase awareness of the mind-body relationship. Remember to pay attention to your thoughts, emotions, and inner feelings while moving. This comprehensive approach unleashes the transforming potential of these activities.

Giving Up Too Soon.

Change does not happen overnight, so be patient with yourself as you learn this new way of moving and being. If you have difficulties or feel like you are not making progress, fight the temptation to give up. Stick with it, and believe that with constant practice, the rewards will begin to emerge.

Remember that the path of somatic exercises is very personal, and the key to success is approaching it with self-compassion, curiosity, and a desire to learn. By recognizing and resolving these frequent beginner errors, you'll be well on your way to realizing the transformational potential of these practices and creating a deeper, more embodied feeling of well-being.

Tips for Consistency and Motivation

As a newcomer discovering somatic exercises, maintaining consistency and motivation might be one of the most difficult tasks. It's easy to become excited and then struggle to maintain a consistent practice. However, with the correct mentality and tactics, you may overcome these challenges and get the transforming advantages of these activities.

Establish a routine.

One key to consistency is to set aside time and space for your somatic exercises. Whether it's a morning ritual or an evening wind-down, aim to make them a must-have component of your daily routine. This will help your body and mind identify the time with the activity, making it easier to continue.

Start small.

If the prospect of a protracted somatic session seems frightening, begin with only a few minutes daily. Even a little 5-10 minute practice can significantly influence your well-being. As you develop the habit, gradually extend the length, but don't feel compelled to go in headlong.

Find What Resonates.

Somatic exercises take numerous forms, ranging from mild stretches to more vigorous motions. Experiment with different techniques to see which ones connect with you. Maintaining motivation and consistency is much simpler when you like the process.

Celebrate Small Wins.

Progress in somatic exercises might be modest, so it's crucial to recognize even the slightest successes. Consider how your body feels after a practice or how your awareness and mindfulness have progressed. Recognizing these small improvements might give a much-needed jolt of inspiration.

Seek Support Having a supportive community may make a huge impact. Join online forums, discover local somatic exercise groups, or seek the advice of a qualified practitioner. Sharing your experience with others may bring accountability, motivation, and a feeling of community that can help you maintain your practice.

Embrace the Journey

Remember that bodily exercises aim to embrace the trip rather than arrive at a certain destination. Approach each exercise with curiosity, self-compassion, and a desire to learn. Trust that the advantages will come in their own time, and enjoy the process of strengthening your mind-body connection.

By following these suggestions, you may develop the consistency and motivation required to make somatic exercises a permanent part of your life. Accept the obstacles, appreciate the tiny victories, and believe that the transforming potential of these practices will continue to emerge, one step at a time.

Modifications for Different Fitness Levels

You may ask how these practices might be tailored to your fitness level and capabilities. The beauty of somatic exercises is their adaptability and accessibility, which allows people of different ages and physical levels to receive the advantages. Whether you're an experienced athlete or just starting on your health path, there are adaptations and changes to ensure that each exercise is safe, pleasant, and successful.

For the physically fit.

If you're already in great physical shape, you might find that some of the fundamental somatic exercises are too simple or unchallenging. However, resist the impulse to overwork oneself or add excessive complication. Remember that the essential strength of these practices is in the quality of your movements and the depth of your awareness, not in their intensity.

One technique to adapt somatic exercises for the physically healthy is to include more dynamic motions or resistance. For example, during the "Leg Swings" exercise, you may extend your range of motion or add a tiny jump after each swing. Alternatively, during the "Shoulder Rolls," you might carry a modest weight in each hand to work the muscles.

Another alternative is to try more advanced somatic techniques that emphasize balance, agility, or coordination. These exercises can help you maintain and perhaps increase your physical fitness while focusing on the mind-body connection important to somatic practice.

For People With Limited Mobility

If you have physical limitations or are recuperating from an accident, you should undertake somatic exercises with caution and thought. However, do not be discouraged by these problems; several adjustments and adaptations are available to guarantee that you continue to benefit from these transforming activities.

One strategy is to concentrate on the parts of your body that are the most movable and accessible. For example, if you have restricted leg mobility, you might focus your practice on the upper body and core. Seated or laying exercises can be especially beneficial for those with restricted mobility because they provide a secure platform and lessen the likelihood of falling or losing balance.

Another crucial factor is to employ props and assistance equipment where necessary. Chairs, walls, and floors may offer support and stability, allowing you to walk confidently and easily. Pillows, blankets, and yoga blocks can adjust positions or add cushioning.

For All Levels.

Regardless of your fitness level or physical ability, the most essential thing is to approach your somatic practice with patience, self-compassion, and a desire to learn. Remember that everyone's body is different, so what works for one person may not work for another. Trust your instincts, listen to your body, and make modifications as required.

By accepting the concepts of bodily exercises and tailoring them to your requirements, you may tap into their transformational potential and build a deeper, more embodied feeling of well-being. Accept the journey, appreciate your accomplishments, and reap the numerous advantages of moving with awareness and intention.

> "Forget the gym, find your flow. Somatic Exercise for Beginners invites you to listen to your body, move with kindness, and celebrate the power within."

CHAPTER 7

Integrating Somatic Awareness into Daily Life

As a novice exploring bodily exercise, you may ask how these practices might be tailored to your fitness level and capabilities. The beauty of somatic exercises is their adaptability and accessibility, which allows people of different ages and physical levels to receive the advantages. Whether you're an experienced athlete or just starting on your health path, there are adaptations and changes to ensure that each exercise is safe, pleasant, and successful.

For the physically fit.

If you're already in great physical shape, you might find that some of the fundamental somatic exercises are too simple or unchallenging. However, resist the impulse to overwork oneself or add excessive complication. Remember that the essential strength of these practices is in the quality of your movements and the depth of your awareness, not in their intensity. One technique to adapt somatic exercises for the physically healthy is to include more dynamic motions or resistance. For example, during the "Leg Swings" exercise, you may extend your range of motion or add a tiny jump after each swing. Alternatively, during the "Shoulder Rolls," you might carry a modest weight in each hand to work the muscles.

Another alternative is to try more advanced somatic techniques that emphasize balance, agility, or coordination. These exercises can help you maintain and perhaps increase your physical fitness while focusing on the mind-body connection important to somatic practice.

For People with Limited Mobility

If you have physical limitations or are recuperating from an accident, you should undertake somatic exercises with caution and thought. However, do not be discouraged by these problems; several adjustments and adaptations are available to guarantee that you continue to benefit from these transforming activities.

One strategy is to concentrate on the parts of your body that are the most movable and accessible. For example, if you have restricted leg mobility, you might focus your practice on the upper body and core. Seated or laying exercises can be especially beneficial for those with restricted mobility because they provide a secure platform and lessen the likelihood of falling or losing balance.

Another crucial factor is to employ props and assistance equipment where necessary. Chairs, walls, and floors may offer support and stability, allowing you to walk confidently and easily. Pillows, blankets, and yoga blocks can adjust positions or add cushioning.

For All Levels.

Regardless of your fitness level or physical ability, the most essential thing is to approach your somatic practice with patience, self-compassion, and a desire to learn. Remember that everyone's body is different, so what works for one person may not work for another. Trust your instincts, listen to your body, and make modifications as required.

By accepting the concepts of bodily exercises and tailoring them to your requirements, you may tap into their transformational potential and build a deeper, more embodied feeling of well-being. Accept the journey, appreciate your accomplishments, and reap the numerous advantages of moving with awareness and intention.

Tracking Progress and Setting Goals

Somatic exercise may feel incredible: a deep breath after a hard day, a sensation of relaxation in your body that you haven't felt in years. However, sometimes improvement might be subtle. We all want that "Aha!" moment, that sudden sense of being a yoga master (or flexibility champion!). The fact is that somatic exercise is more of a trek than a sprint. It's about enjoying the trip, seeing the minor changes along the way, and appreciating the accomplishments that get you to the summit.

So, how do we follow this particular path?

- ❖ Locate your "feel-good" meter. Instead of focusing on the numbers on the scale, consider how your body feels. Does the persistent ache in your lower back seem to subside after a few sessions? Can you finally reach your toes (without feeling like you're going to fall over!)? These tiny successes indicate that you're on the correct course.

- ❖ Keep a basic journal. Take a few notes after each session. How did you feel before, during, and after? Did you find a new exercise that felt very liberating? These notes become a treasure trove, reminding you of how far you've gone on days when motivation is low.

- ❖ Celebrate, not conquer: Achieving a particular position or mastering a difficult sequence is amazing! But don't forget to enjoy the small things. Maybe you were finally able to sit comfortably for the full meditation session, or maybe you just turned up to your mat when you didn't feel like it. All of these accomplishments need to be recognized.

Remember that somatic exercise is a process of self-discovery. Tracking your progress and creating objectives that are meaningful to you will provide you with the incentive to continue exploring, as well as the delight of feeling your body move and breathe freely again.

Effective ways to set achievable goals for beginners in somatic exercises

Here are some excellent strategies for creating realistic objectives for beginners in somatic exercises:

- **Set specific and measurable goals:** When defining goals, make them as explicit as possible. Vague goals such as "improve flexibility" are more difficult to measure. Set quantifiable objectives, such as "increase range of motion in my hamstrings by 10 degrees" or "be able to hold a seated forward fold for 1 minute without discomfort."
- **Focus on Process, Not Just Results:** With somatic exercises, the act of tuning into your body's sensations and moving deliberately is just as crucial as the outcome. Set goals for growing body awareness, lowering stress, and nurturing a sense of ease, rather than merely physical improvements.
- **Begin small and build up:** As a newbie, set small, attainable goals first. "Practice somatic exercises 3 times per week for 10-15 minutes" or "notice 3 new body sensations during each practice" are excellent beginning points. You may raise the difficulty as you gain consistency.
- **Celebrate incremental progress:** Somatic changes might be modest, so note and applaud even minor victories. Notice when you feel more grounded, when a movement feels smoother, or when you can focus for longer periods of time. Maintaining a notebook can aid in tracking these small changes.
- **Align goals with your values:** Consider what matters most to you: pain relief, posture improvement, or stress management. Align your goals with your own beliefs and needs to stay motivated.

- **Be flexible and adjust as needed:** Your goals may need to change as you advance. Check in with yourself on a frequent basis, and don't be hesitant to adjust your objectives if something isn't working or your requirements change.

The idea is to begin basic, focus on the process, and enjoy tiny victories. With patience and perseverance, you may gradually progress towards more ambitious somatic objectives.

Setting SMART Goals for Your Somatic Practice

As a newcomer to the transforming realm of somatic exercises, having clear and attainable goals may be a game changer. By using the SMART framework (Specific, Measurable, Achievable, Relevant, and Time-bound), you may design a road map for success that will keep you motivated, engaged, and thrilled about your progress.

Specific

When it comes to somatic practice, nonspecific goals like "improve my flexibility" or "reduce stress" might be difficult to quantify and attain. Instead, try to be as specific as possible. A possible goal is to "increase the range of motion in your hamstrings by 10 degrees" and/or "be able to hold a seated forward fold for 1 minute without discomfort." The more exact you can be, the easier it will be to monitor your progress.

Measurable

Quantifying your objectives is critical because it helps you to measure your progress over time. Having tangible metrics to assess, whether it's the number of somatic exercises you do each week, the length of your practice, or the changes in your bodily sensations, can offer you a distinct feeling of achievement and keep you motivated.

Achievable

Set objectives that challenge you but do not overwhelm or discourage you. As a novice, set small, incremental goals that you may reasonably achieve with persistent effort. This will boost your confidence and momentum, opening the door for more ambitious goals in the future.

Relevant

Your somatic objectives should be intimately related to your own beliefs, needs, and general well-being. Perhaps you want to lessen chronic pain, enhance your posture, or develop a stronger feeling of mind-body connection. Whatever your motives, be sure your objectives are important and applicable to your life.

Time-bound

Setting a schedule for your objectives may give you a feeling of organization and urgency, allowing you to stay focused and accountable. Whether it's a weekly, monthly, or quarterly goal, having a clear deadline will give your practice direction and drive.

As you go on this sensory adventure, remember to be patient, kind, and open to adjust. Your goals may change over time, and that's absolutely OK. The goal is to stay focused, appreciate your achievements, and believe that the transforming advantages of these practices will continue to emerge, one step at a time.

Tracking Your Progress and Celebrating Milestones

As you begin your somatic exercise adventure, measuring your progress and celebrating your accomplishments is critical. This helps you stay motivated, acknowledge your achievements, and strengthen your mind-body connection.

Tracking Progress

Keep a notebook or log of your somatic exercises, noting how you feel before and after each one. Pay attention to any changes in your physical, mental, or emotional state. This allows you to spot patterns, track your progress, and change your practice as necessary.

Celebrating Milestones

Take time to recognize your accomplishments when you reach new milestones. Recognize your tiny wins, such as finishing a new activity or seeing a specific improvement. This might be as basic as a mental high-five or a quick expression of thanks.

Feeling the progress

As you track your progress, you may notice small shifts in your body and mind. Perhaps you feel more stable, flexible, or calm. These transitions may be powerful and transformational, and identifying them can help you stay focused on your practice.

Staying motivated

Tracking your progress and celebrating milestones helps you stay motivated and interested. You see actual results for your efforts, which may be a tremendous motivation. This helps you maintain consistency and commitment to your somatic workout routine.

Remember that the journey of somatic exercises is unique to each individual, and improvement will seem different. Tracking your progress and enjoying milestones will help you stay focused, motivated, and connected to your body and mind.

Expanding Your Knowledge

As someone new discovering the realm of somatic exercises, you may feel excited and curious about the many possibilities that await you. As you explore further into these transformational activities, you will realize that there is always more to learn and discover. Embracing this perspective of constant development and discovery may be the key to realizing the full potential of your somatic experience.

One of the most enjoyable parts of learning somatic exercises is the chance to strengthen your mind-body connection. With each new technique or approach you try, you'll discover new levels of self-awareness, including subtle feelings and patterns you may have noticed before. This increased feeling of embodied consciousness may be genuinely life-changing, allowing you to move, feel, and live more freely and purposefully. Perhaps you'll be drawn to Tai Chi's smooth, flowing motions or the contemplative aspects of Qigong. Perhaps you'll discover the power of breathwork and how it can significantly improve your mental and physical well-being. Alternatively, you may explore the realm of yoga, marveling at how these ancient practices can improve your flexibility, strength, and general sense of balance.

Don't be scared to push yourself beyond your comfort zone as you broaden your knowledge. Attend classes, consult with skilled practitioners, and immerse yourself in the rich tapestry of somatic traditions from across the world. Each new encounter will provide a distinct viewpoint, encouraging you to approach your practice with an open mind and want to learn.

Remember that the goal of somatic exercises is to embrace the process of constant growth and self-discovery rather than to arrive at a particular destination. Celebrate your accomplishments, accept your limits, and believe that with each new step, you will get a better awareness of yourself and the vast wisdom that lives inside your body.

So, let your curiosity guide you and begin on a lifelong journey to discover the transformational potential of somatic exercise. The more you understand, the more you'll see that the possibilities are genuinely limitless.

Conclusion

Somatic exercise is more than just stretching and maintaining good posture. It's about reconnecting with your body, respecting its individual requirements, and discovering a sense of well-being that goes well beyond the mat. SOMATIC EXERCISE FOR BEGINNERS is your guide to this transforming journey. With straightforward instructions, entertaining exercises, and a focus on mindfulness, this book will help you regain your body's inherent potential.

Do not wait for the illusive "perfect time" to start. Your body is ready now. Order your copy of SOMATIC EXERCISE FOR BEGINNERS today and start on the path to a more connected, powerful self.

And, to help others discover the benefits of somatic exercise, we respectfully request that you give an honest review after reading the book. Your ideas will be important to future readers, and together we can build a community that values mindful movement and self-discovery.

www.ingramcontent.com/pod-product-compliance
Lightning Source LLC
Chambersburg PA
CBHW071950210526
45479CB00003B/875